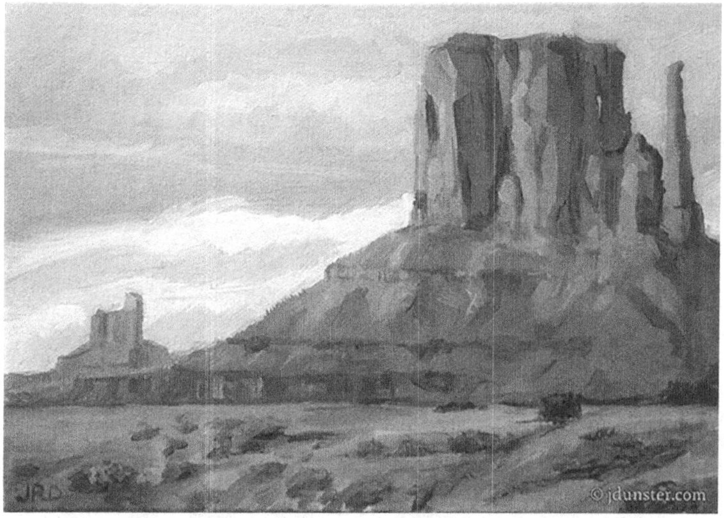

Six-Month Kidney-Friendly & CKD Food Journal

& Daily Planner

NAME: ....

CONTACT INFO: ....

DATE STARTED: ....

DATE ENDED: ....

EMERGENCY CONTACT: ....

Green Verdugo Studio

greenverdugostudio.com

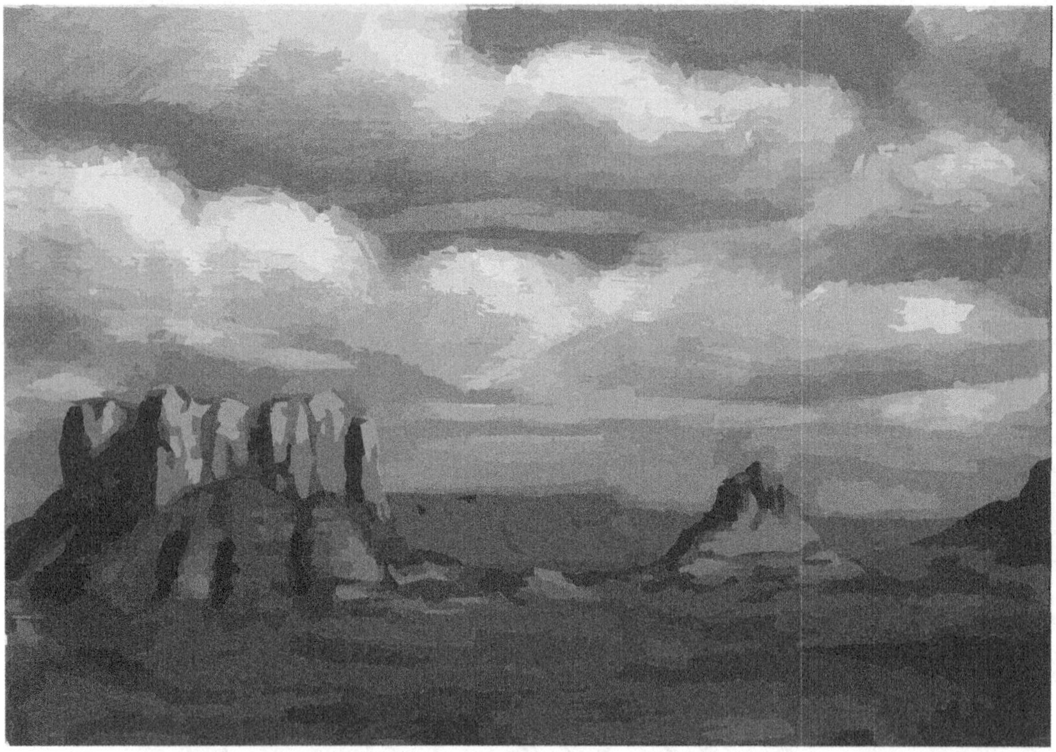

Green Verdugo Press
gverdugo.com
ISBN: 978-0-9977518-0-2

HIGH ALKALINE, LOW-ACID DIET JOURNAL

This journal is designed to assist the kidney patient in keeping track of the important food values from their daily diet, such as fluid intake, as well as calories, fat, protein, potassium, phosphorus, sodium, PRAL numbers and fiber. (PRAL stands for "potential renal acid load" and foods higher in acid-producing elements—like meats and dairy—are harder on the kidneys.) There's also a blank box for adding an additional value that is significant for the individual patient. **The diary should last for six months if used daily.** There is also an added "daily schedule/planner" section at the bottom half of each page. Its use is optional.

WHAT IS PRAL?

Most of us know what protein, potassium and phosphorus are likely to be tracked by CKD patients, but what is PRAL, exactly, and how does it work?

Simply put, each food has its own PRAL "number." Food with a positive number (for instance, +3) is more acid-producing for the body and thus harder on the kidneys. Negative number foods (-3) are alkaline-producing (better for the kidneys). The goal is to tally up all the numbers of everything eaten during the day and make sure the final total is a negative number. A total in the negative numbers means that, on average, the food eaten that day was alkaline-producing and therefore, more protective of the kidneys.

Generally, plants (fruits and veggies) have negative (alkaline) numbers while animal-based foods and dairy have positive (acid) numbers. Grains often have positive numbers, but much lower in comparison to animal-based foods.

Keeping track of PRAL numbers may lead to some kidney patients avoiding all animal-based foods, while others will limit their intake of meats and dairy but not eliminate these foods completely. This will be a personal decision and should be discussed with your doctor and/or nutritionist.

This kidney dietitian's site gives an excellent explanation of the benefits of PRAL: **https://www.thekidneydietitian.org/pral/** Please read this site and do other research to better understand PRAL for CKD.

This medical study explains more about "dietary acid load" and gives some of the reasons why a diet rich in plant-based foods could be a good idea for kidney disease patients. **https://www.ncbi.nlm.nih.gov/pmc/articles/PMC6627351/**

"Metabolic acidosis in chronic kidney disease (CKD) is aggravated by the high consumption of meat and refined cereals, increasing the dietary acid load, while the intake of fruit and vegetables is able to neutralize the acidosis and its deleterious consequences. Phosphorus absorption and bioavailability is also lower in a vegetarian diet, reducing hyperphosphatemia, a known cause of cardiovascular mortality in CKD." (A small excerpt from this report.)

This medical study: **https://pubmed.ncbi.nlm.nih.gov/33075387/** states: *"It is likely that the risks for both issues may not have been as significant as previously thought, while the advantages are vast. In conclusion, the risk to benefit ratio of plant-based diets appears to be tilting in favor of their more prevalent use."*

USEFUL RESOURCES & LINKS:

Kidneyhood.com: Website for author Lee Hull's popular book about how to fight kidney disease. The companion cookbook is mostly plant-based.

Dadvice TV (YouTube channel): Many helpful and encouraging videos about diet, and other techniques to help you live well with kidney disease.

DietGrail.com: Look for the link to the "low acid diet/alkaline diet" database to see the PRAL values for many foods.

AJKD.org: American Journal of Kidney Diseases site. Look for "KDQOI" 2020 Guideline for Nutrition. They now emphasize and encourage a diet that is mainly plant-based.

THE WAY OF EATING IN A NUTSHELL

Various popular CKD-friendly diets share a few things in common, which you can find online and/or in books. (This list isn't definitive or complete and isn't intended to be medical advice.)

- Eating mostly whole foods & avoiding processed, refined or fast foods.
- Limited or no refined sugar, moderate or no added oils. Other sweeteners like stevia or maple syrup might be used.
- The diet often consists of mostly vegetables and fruits. Grains and legumes are usually permitted but in more measured amounts. Animal products like beef, chicken, fish, eggs, milk and cheese may not allowed, or will be limited.
- Eat gluten-free and use caution with soy. Certain CKD patients might want to avoid "Eveningshade" vegetables like potatoes and tomatoes.
- This way of eating is for health only and NOT philosophical or political. Some CKD patients may occasionally consume animal flesh. Nobody is pushing any vegetarian/vegan agenda here! The stronger emphasis on more plants in the diet is backed up by many medical studies.
- Some people may see marked improvement when they improve their diet, but if they return to their "old" way of eating, the problems return. The secret may be to keep eating this way even when things get better.
- For those struggling to adjust to a diet with a strong plant-based emphasis, the advice is to make gradual changes. It does get better and the results are worth it.
- People with early/mild CKD will also benefit from this diet. It's never too soon to start preserving kidney function and preventing decline!

HOW TO USE THE JOURNAL

Log all your meals and snacks to keep track of your calories, fat, protein, potassium, phosphorus, sodium, PRAL, and fiber. This will help you maintain your kidney-friendly diet.

The abbreviations in the journal:

cal: calories **fat:** fat in grams **pro:** protein in grams **pot:** potassium **pho:** phosphorus **sod:** sodium **PRAL:** Potential Renal Acid Load (see previous pages for an explanation about this and why it's important to many kidney disease patients to keep track of their PRAL numbers). **fib:** fiber

The food value numbers (you'll see some examples of these on the next page) are in the most commonly used units seen on food labels. (For example, fat is measured in grams, as is protein, so it is assumed that the number "2" in the fat or protein column refers to 2 grams. A number of 100 in the sodium column would mean 100 milligrams, and so forth and so on.)

There is one extra space to list values for whatever else is important to you. At the bottom there is more space to add additional details about the day, reminders, appointments, memories, or whatever!

There is room to check off an intake of up to twelve 8-oz. units of fluid, but this does not imply that you must or should drink this amount of water or fluid daily. (A common recommendation is eight glasses a day, but this can vary for each individual.) There is also space to record your weight—but it probably isn't necessary to do this daily.

EVERYONE'S SITUATION IS UNIQUE

Don't feel like you must fill out every food value. It depends on what is needed for your particular diet. Listen to your doctor's or nutritionist's opinions and guidance. Each CKD patient has different lab results and their diet can be tailored around their unique dietary needs. For example, some patients might have to limit potassium intake, while others won't have any restrictions at all. One size does not fit all when it comes to a kidney-friendly diet!

DON'T FREAK OUT ABOUT OVER POSSIBLE DIETARY CHANGES

Just go little by little. Many CKD patients have seen great improvements in their labs by switching to a plant-rich diet. This doesn't mean that you can't ever enjoy a burger or steak again. With any health challege there is a period of adjustment. New recipes will be learned. New habits will take time to be formed. Your future is what's most important and you will soon learn to embrace the changes that benefit your health.

SAMPLE FOOD VALUES LIST

(This list is NOT meant to represent the best foods or the most popular foods for every kidney disease patient.

Values are an estimation and may not always be completely accurate.)

FRUITS & VEGGIES

Apple, med: Cal 90, Fat 0, Pro 0, Pot 200, Phos 20, Sod 0, PRAL -3, fib 4
Avocado, one mini or half of a regular size: Cal 160, Fat 16, Pro 2, Pot 300, Phos 30, Sod 0, PRAL -8, Fib 4.6
Broccoli florets, cooked, 1 cup: Cal 25, Fat 0, Pro 3, Pot 280, Phos 30, Sod 15, PRAL -1, fib 3
Carrot, 1 med: Cal 25, Fat 0, Pro 0.5, Pot 200, Pho 20, Sod 45, PRAL -3, Fib 2
Celery, two stalks: Cal 20, Fat 0, Pro 1, Pot 330, Phos 30, Sod 110, PRAL -7, fib 2

LEGUMES & GRAINS:

Rice, white, 1/4 cup dry: Cal 160, Fat 0, Pro 3, Pot 40, Pho 50, Sod 0, PRAL +2, Fib 0
Rice, brown, 1/4 cup dry: Cal 160, Fat 1, Pro 3, Pot 60, Pho 90, Sod 0, PRAL +2.5, Fib 1
Brown Lentils, 1/4 cup dry: Cal 160, Fat 0, Pro 9, Pot 500, Pho 250, Sod 0, PRAL +5, Fib 9

MY FAVORITE FOOD VALUES LIST

MY FAVORITE FOOD VALUES LIST

DATE .... weight ....

cups of fluid:

Food eaten	cal	fat	pro	pot	pho	sod	PRAL	fib	
TOTALS									

√	→	TO DO & TASK LIST

Hour	Schedule

Events of the day: ....

DATE .... weight ....

cups of fluid:

Food eaten	cal	fat	pro	pot	pho	sod	PRAL	fib	
TOTALS									

√	→	TO DO & TASK LIST

Hour	Schedule

Events of the day: ....

DATE

weight

cups of fluid:

Food eaten	cal	fat	pro	pot	pho	sod	PRAL	fib	
TOTALS									

√	→	TO DO & TASK LIST

Hour	Schedule

Events of the day:

DATE .... weight ....

cups of fluid:

Food eaten	cal	fat	pro	pot	pho	sod	PRAL	fib	
TOTALS									

√	→	TO DO & TASK LIST

Hour	Schedule

Events of the day: ....

....

....

....

DATE .... weight ....

cups of fluid:

Food eaten	cal	fat	pro	pot	pho	sod	PRAL	fib	
TOTALS									

√	→	TO DO & TASK LIST

Hour	Schedule

Events of the day: ....

DATE .... weight ....

cups of fluid:

Food eaten	cal	fat	pro	pot	pho	sod	PRAL	fib	
TOTALS									

√	→	TO DO & TASK LIST

Hour	Schedule

Events of the day: ....

DATE

weight

cups of fluid:

Food eaten	cal	fat	pro	pot	pho	sod	PRAL	fib	
TOTALS									

√	→	TO DO & TASK LIST

Hour	Schedule

Events of the day:

DATE .... weight ....

cups of fluid:

Food eaten	cal	fat	pro	pot	pho	sod	PRAL	fib	
TOTALS									

√	→	TO DO & TASK LIST

Hour	Schedule

Events of the day: ....

DATE .... weight ....

cups of fluid:

Food eaten	cal	fat	pro	pot	pho	sod	PRAL	fib	
TOTALS									

√	→	TO DO & TASK LIST

Hour	Schedule

Events of the day: ....

DATE .... weight ....

cups of fluid:

Food eaten	cal	fat	pro	pot	pho	sod	PRAL	fib	
TOTALS									

√	→	TO DO & TASK LIST

Hour	Schedule

Events of the day: ....

....

....

....

DATE .... weight ....

cups of fluid:

Food eaten	cal	fat	pro	pot	pho	sod	PRAL	fib	
TOTALS									

√	→	TO DO & TASK LIST

Hour	Schedule

Events of the day: ....

DATE .... weight ....

cups of fluid:

Food eaten	cal	fat	pro	pot	pho	sod	PRAL	fib	
TOTALS									

√	→	TO DO & TASK LIST

Hour	Schedule

Events of the day: ....

DATE .... weight ....

cups of fluid:

Food eaten	cal	fat	pro	pot	pho	sod	PRAL	fib	
TOTALS									

√	→	TO DO & TASK LIST

Hour	Schedule

Events of the day: ....

DATE .... weight ....

cups of fluid:

Food eaten	cal	fat	pro	pot	pho	sod	PRAL	fib	
TOTALS									

√	→	TO DO & TASK LIST

Hour	Schedule

Events of the day: ....

DATE .... weight ....

cups of fluid:

Food eaten	cal	fat	pro	pot	pho	sod	PRAL	fib	
TOTALS									

√	→	TO DO & TASK LIST

Hour	Schedule

Events of the day: ....

DATE .... weight ....

cups of fluid:

Food eaten	cal	fat	pro	pot	pho	sod	PRAL	fib	
TOTALS									

√	→	TO DO & TASK LIST

Hour	Schedule

Events of the day: ....

DATE .... weight ....

cups of fluid:

Food eaten	cal	fat	pro	pot	pho	sod	PRAL	fib	
TOTALS									

√	→	TO DO & TASK LIST

Hour	Schedule

Events of the day: ....

DATE .... weight ....

cups of fluid:

Food eaten	cal	fat	pro	pot	pho	sod	PRAL	fib	
TOTALS									

√	→	TO DO & TASK LIST

Hour	Schedule

Events of the day: ....

DATE .... weight ....

cups of fluid:

Food eaten	cal	fat	pro	pot	pho	sod	PRAL	fib	
TOTALS									

√	→	TO DO & TASK LIST

Hour	Schedule

Events of the day: ....

....

....

....

DATE .... weight ....

cups of fluid:

Food eaten	cal	fat	pro	pot	pho	sod	PRAL	fib	
TOTALS									

√	→	TO DO & TASK LIST

Hour	Schedule

Events of the day: ....

....

....

....

DATE .... weight ....

cups of fluid:

Food eaten	cal	fat	pro	pot	pho	sod	PRAL	fib	
TOTALS									

√	→	TO DO & TASK LIST

Hour	Schedule

Events of the day: ....

DATE .... weight ....

cups of fluid:

Food eaten	cal	fat	pro	pot	pho	sod	PRAL	fib	
TOTALS									

√	→	TO DO & TASK LIST

Hour	Schedule

Events of the day: ....

DATE .... weight ....

cups of fluid:

Food eaten	cal	fat	pro	pot	pho	sod	PRAL	fib	
TOTALS									

√	→	TO DO & TASK LIST

Hour	Schedule

Events of the day: ....

DATE .... weight ....

cups of fluid:

Food eaten	cal	fat	pro	pot	pho	sod	PRAL	fib	
TOTALS									

√	→	TO DO & TASK LIST

Hour	Schedule

Events of the day: ....

DATE .... weight ....

cups of fluid:

Food eaten	cal	fat	pro	pot	pho	sod	PRAL	fib	
TOTALS									

√	→	TO DO & TASK LIST

Hour	Schedule

Events of the day: ....

DATE .... weight ....

cups of fluid:

Food eaten	cal	fat	pro	pot	pho	sod	PRAL	fib	
TOTALS									

√	→	TO DO & TASK LIST

Hour	Schedule

Events of the day: ....

DATE .... weight ....

cups of fluid:

Food eaten	cal	fat	pro	pot	pho	sod	PRAL	fib	
TOTALS									

√	→	TO DO & TASK LIST

Hour	Schedule

Events of the day: ....

DATE .... weight ....

cups of fluid:

Food eaten	cal	fat	pro	pot	pho	sod	PRAL	fib	
TOTALS									

√	→	TO DO & TASK LIST

Hour	Schedule

Events of the day: ....

DATE .... weight ....

cups of fluid:

Food eaten	cal	fat	pro	pot	pho	sod	PRAL	fib	
TOTALS									

√	→	TO DO & TASK LIST

Hour	Schedule

Events of the day: ....

DATE .... weight ....

cups of fluid:

Food eaten	cal	fat	pro	pot	pho	sod	PRAL	fib	
TOTALS									

√	→	TO DO & TASK LIST

Hour	Schedule

Events of the day: ....

....

....

....

DATE .... weight ....

cups of fluid:

Food eaten	cal	fat	pro	pot	pho	sod	PRAL	fib	
TOTALS									

√	→	TO DO & TASK LIST

Hour	Schedule

Events of the day: ....

DATE .... weight ....

cups of fluid:

Food eaten	cal	fat	pro	pot	pho	sod	PRAL	fib	
TOTALS									

√	→	TO DO & TASK LIST

Hour	Schedule

Events of the day: ....

DATE .... weight ....

cups of fluid:

Food eaten	cal	fat	pro	pot	pho	sod	PRAL	fib	
TOTALS									

√	→	TO DO & TASK LIST

Hour	Schedule

Events of the day: ....

DATE .... weight ....

cups of fluid:

Food eaten	cal	fat	pro	pot	pho	sod	PRAL	fib	
TOTALS									

√	→	TO DO & TASK LIST

Hour	Schedule

Events of the day: ....

DATE .... weight ....

cups of fluid:

Food eaten	cal	fat	pro	pot	pho	sod	PRAL	fib	
TOTALS									

√	→	TO DO & TASK LIST

Hour	Schedule

Events of the day: ....

DATE .... weight ....

cups of fluid:

Food eaten	cal	fat	pro	pot	pho	sod	PRAL	fib	
TOTALS									

√	→	TO DO & TASK LIST

Hour	Schedule

Events of the day: ....

....

....

....

DATE .... weight ....

cups of fluid:

Food eaten	cal	fat	pro	pot	pho	sod	PRAL	fib	
TOTALS									

√	→	TO DO & TASK LIST

Hour	Schedule

Events of the day: ....

DATE .... weight ....

cups of fluid:

Food eaten	cal	fat	pro	pot	pho	sod	PRAL	fib	
TOTALS									

√	→	TO DO & TASK LIST

Hour	Schedule

Events of the day: ....

DATE .... weight ....

cups of fluid:

Food eaten	cal	fat	pro	pot	pho	sod	PRAL	fib	
TOTALS									

√	→	TO DO & TASK LIST

Hour	Schedule

Events of the day: ....

DATE .... weight ....

cups of fluid:

Food eaten	cal	fat	pro	pot	pho	sod	PRAL	fib	
TOTALS									

√	→	TO DO & TASK LIST

Hour	Schedule

Events of the day: ....

DATE .... weight ....

cups of fluid:

Food eaten	cal	fat	pro	pot	pho	sod	PRAL	fib	
TOTALS									

√	→	TO DO & TASK LIST

Hour	Schedule

Events of the day: ....

DATE .... weight ....

cups of fluid:

Food eaten	cal	fat	pro	pot	pho	sod	PRAL	fib	
TOTALS									

√	→	TO DO & TASK LIST

Hour	Schedule

Events of the day: ....

DATE .... weight ....

cups of fluid:

Food eaten	cal	fat	pro	pot	pho	sod	PRAL	fib	
TOTALS									

√	→	TO DO & TASK LIST

Hour	Schedule

Events of the day: ....

....

....

....

DATE .... weight ....

cups of fluid:

Food eaten	cal	fat	pro	pot	pho	sod	PRAL	fib	
TOTALS									

√	→	TO DO & TASK LIST

Hour	Schedule

Events of the day: ....

DATE .... weight ....

cups of fluid:

Food eaten	cal	fat	pro	pot	pho	sod	PRAL	fib	
TOTALS									

√	→	TO DO & TASK LIST

Hour	Schedule

Events of the day: ....

DATE .... weight ....

cups of fluid:

Food eaten	cal	fat	pro	pot	pho	sod	PRAL	fib	
TOTALS									

√	→	TO DO & TASK LIST

Hour	Schedule

Events of the day: ....

DATE .... weight ....

cups of fluid:

Food eaten	cal	fat	pro	pot	pho	sod	PRAL	fib	
TOTALS									

√	→	TO DO & TASK LIST

Hour	Schedule

Events of the day: ....

DATE .... weight ....

cups of fluid:

Food eaten	cal	fat	pro	pot	pho	sod	PRAL	fib	
TOTALS									

√	→	TO DO & TASK LIST

Hour	Schedule

Events of the day: ....

....

....

....

DATE .... weight ....

cups of fluid:

Food eaten	cal	fat	pro	pot	pho	sod	PRAL	fib	
TOTALS									

√	→	TO DO & TASK LIST

Hour	Schedule

Events of the day: ....

DATE .... weight ....

cups of fluid:

Food eaten	cal	fat	pro	pot	pho	sod	PRAL	fib	
TOTALS									

√	→	TO DO & TASK LIST

Hour	Schedule

Events of the day: ....

DATE .... weight ....

cups of fluid:

Food eaten	cal	fat	pro	pot	pho	sod	PRAL	fib	
TOTALS									

√	→	TO DO & TASK LIST

Hour	Schedule

Events of the day: ....

....

....

....

DATE .... weight ....

cups of fluid:

Food eaten	cal	fat	pro	pot	pho	sod	PRAL	fib	
TOTALS									

√	→	TO DO & TASK LIST

Hour	Schedule

Events of the day: ....

....

....

....

DATE .... weight ....

cups of fluid:

Food eaten	cal	fat	pro	pot	pho	sod	PRAL	fib	
TOTALS									

√	→	TO DO & TASK LIST

Hour	Schedule

Events of the day: ....

DATE ………………………… weight …………

cups of fluid:

Food eaten	cal	fat	pro	pot	pho	sod	PRAL	fib	
TOTALS									

√	→	TO DO & TASK LIST

Hour	Schedule

Events of the day: …………………………

DATE .... weight ....

cups of fluid:

Food eaten	cal	fat	pro	pot	pho	sod	PRAL	fib	
TOTALS									

√	→	TO DO & TASK LIST

Hour	Schedule

Events of the day: ....

....

....

....

DATE .... weight ....

cups of fluid:

Food eaten	cal	fat	pro	pot	pho	sod	PRAL	fib	
TOTALS									

√	→	TO DO & TASK LIST

Hour	Schedule

Events of the day: ....

....

....

....

DATE ________________ weight ________

cups of fluid:

Food eaten	cal	fat	pro	pot	pho	sod	PRAL	fib	
TOTALS									

√	→	TO DO & TASK LIST

Hour	Schedule

Events of the day: ________________

DATE .... weight ....

cups of fluid:

Food eaten	cal	fat	pro	pot	pho	sod	PRAL	fib	
TOTALS									

√	→	TO DO & TASK LIST

Hour	Schedule

Events of the day: ....

DATE .... weight ....

cups of fluid:

Food eaten	cal	fat	pro	pot	pho	sod	PRAL	fib	
TOTALS									

√	→	TO DO & TASK LIST

Hour	Schedule

Events of the day: ....

....

....

....

DATE .... weight ....

cups of fluid:

Food eaten	cal	fat	pro	pot	pho	sod	PRAL	fib	
TOTALS									

√	→	TO DO & TASK LIST

Hour	Schedule

Events of the day: ....

....

....

....

DATE ____________ weight ____________

cups of fluid:

Food eaten	cal	fat	pro	pot	pho	sod	PRAL	fib	
TOTALS									

√	→	TO DO & TASK LIST

Hour	Schedule

Events of the day: ____________

DATE .... weight ....

cups of fluid:

Food eaten	cal	fat	pro	pot	pho	sod	PRAL	fib	
TOTALS									

√	→	TO DO & TASK LIST

Hour	Schedule

Events of the day: ....

....

....

....

DATE .... weight ....

cups of fluid:

Food eaten	cal	fat	pro	pot	pho	sod	PRAL	fib	
TOTALS									

√	→	TO DO & TASK LIST

Hour	Schedule

Events of the day: ....

DATE .... weight ....

cups of fluid:

Food eaten	cal	fat	pro	pot	pho	sod	PRAL	fib	
TOTALS									

√	→	TO DO & TASK LIST

Hour	Schedule

Events of the day: ....

....

....

....

DATE .... weight ....

cups of fluid:

Food eaten	cal	fat	pro	pot	pho	sod	PRAL	fib	
TOTALS									

√	→	TO DO & TASK LIST

Hour	Schedule

Events of the day: ....

DATE .... weight ....

cups of fluid:

Food eaten	cal	fat	pro	pot	pho	sod	PRAL	fib	
TOTALS									

√	→	TO DO & TASK LIST

Hour	Schedule

Events of the day: ....

DATE .... weight ....

cups of fluid:

Food eaten	cal	fat	pro	pot	pho	sod	PRAL	fib	
TOTALS									

√	→	TO DO & TASK LIST

Hour	Schedule

Events of the day: ....

DATE .... weight ....

cups of fluid:

Food eaten	cal	fat	pro	pot	pho	sod	PRAL	fib	
TOTALS									

√	→	TO DO & TASK LIST

Hour	Schedule

Events of the day: ....

DATE ______________________ weight __________

cups of fluid:

Food eaten	cal	fat	pro	pot	pho	sod	PRAL	fib	
TOTALS									

√	→	TO DO & TASK LIST

Hour	Schedule

Events of the day: ______________________

DATE .... weight ....

cups of fluid:

Food eaten	cal	fat	pro	pot	pho	sod	PRAL	fib	
TOTALS									

√	→	TO DO & TASK LIST

Hour	Schedule

Events of the day: ....

DATE .... weight ....

cups of fluid:

Food eaten	cal	fat	pro	pot	pho	sod	PRAL	fib	
TOTALS									

√	→	TO DO & TASK LIST

Hour	Schedule

Events of the day: ....

DATE .... weight ....

cups of fluid:

Food eaten	cal	fat	pro	pot	pho	sod	PRAL	fib	
TOTALS									

√	→	TO DO & TASK LIST

Hour	Schedule

Events of the day: ....

DATE .... weight ....

cups of fluid:

Food eaten	cal	fat	pro	pot	pho	sod	PRAL	fib	
TOTALS									

√	→	TO DO & TASK LIST

Hour	Schedule

Events of the day: ....

DATE .... weight ....

cups of fluid:

Food eaten	cal	fat	pro	pot	pho	sod	PRAL	fib	
TOTALS									

√	→	TO DO & TASK LIST

Hour	Schedule

Events of the day: ....

....

....

....

DATE .... weight ....

cups of fluid:

Food eaten	cal	fat	pro	pot	pho	sod	PRAL	fib	
TOTALS									

√	→	TO DO & TASK LIST

Hour	Schedule

Events of the day: ....

DATE .... weight ....

cups of fluid:

Food eaten	cal	fat	pro	pot	pho	sod	PRAL	fib	
TOTALS									

√	→	TO DO & TASK LIST

Hour	Schedule

Events of the day: ....

....

....

....

DATE .... weight ....

cups of fluid:

Food eaten	cal	fat	pro	pot	pho	sod	PRAL	fib	
TOTALS									

√	→	TO DO & TASK LIST

Hour	Schedule

Events of the day: ....

....

....

....

DATE .... weight ....

cups of fluid:

Food eaten	cal	fat	pro	pot	pho	sod	PRAL	fib	
TOTALS									

√	→	TO DO & TASK LIST

Hour	Schedule

Events of the day: ....

....

....

....

DATE .... weight ....

cups of fluid:

Food eaten	cal	fat	pro	pot	pho	sod	PRAL	fib	
TOTALS									

√	→	TO DO & TASK LIST

Hour	Schedule

Events of the day: ....

DATE ________________ weight ________

cups of fluid:

Food eaten	cal	fat	pro	pot	pho	sod	PRAL	fib	
TOTALS									

√	→	TO DO & TASK LIST

Hour	Schedule

Events of the day: ________________

DATE .... weight ....

cups of fluid:

Food eaten	cal	fat	pro	pot	pho	sod	PRAL	fib	
TOTALS									

√	→	TO DO & TASK LIST

Hour	Schedule

Events of the day: ....

....

....

....

DATE .... weight ....

cups of fluid:

Food eaten	cal	fat	pro	pot	pho	sod	PRAL	fib	
TOTALS									

√	→	TO DO & TASK LIST

Hour	Schedule

Events of the day: ....

DATE .... weight ....

cups of fluid:

Food eaten	cal	fat	pro	pot	pho	sod	PRAL	fib	
TOTALS									

√	→	TO DO & TASK LIST

Hour	Schedule

Events of the day: ....

DATE .... weight ....

cups of fluid:

Food eaten	cal	fat	pro	pot	pho	sod	PRAL	fib	
TOTALS									

√	→	TO DO & TASK LIST

Hour	Schedule

Events of the day: ....

....

....

....

DATE .... weight ....

cups of fluid:

Food eaten	cal	fat	pro	pot	pho	sod	PRAL	fib	
TOTALS									

√	→	TO DO & TASK LIST

Hour	Schedule

Events of the day: ....

DATE .... weight ....

cups of fluid:

Food eaten	cal	fat	pro	pot	pho	sod	PRAL	fib	
TOTALS									

√	→	TO DO & TASK LIST

Hour	Schedule

Events of the day: ....

DATE .... weight ....

cups of fluid:

Food eaten	cal	fat	pro	pot	pho	sod	PRAL	fib	
TOTALS									

√	→	TO DO & TASK LIST

Hour	Schedule

Events of the day: ....

DATE .... weight ....

cups of fluid:

Food eaten	cal	fat	pro	pot	pho	sod	PRAL	fib	
TOTALS									

√	→	TO DO & TASK LIST

Hour	Schedule

Events of the day: ....

DATE .... weight ....

cups of fluid:

Food eaten	cal	fat	pro	pot	pho	sod	PRAL	fib	
TOTALS									

√	→	TO DO & TASK LIST

Hour	Schedule

Events of the day: ....

DATE .... weight ....

cups of fluid:

Food eaten	cal	fat	pro	pot	pho	sod	PRAL	fib	
TOTALS									

√	→	TO DO & TASK LIST

Hour	Schedule

Events of the day: ....

DATE .... weight ....

cups of fluid:

Food eaten	cal	fat	pro	pot	pho	sod	PRAL	fib	
TOTALS									

√	→	TO DO & TASK LIST

Hour	Schedule

Events of the day: ....

DATE .... weight ....

cups of fluid:

Food eaten	cal	fat	pro	pot	pho	sod	PRAL	fib	
TOTALS									

√	→	TO DO & TASK LIST

Hour	Schedule

Events of the day: ....

....

....

....

DATE .... weight ....

cups of fluid:

Food eaten	cal	fat	pro	pot	pho	sod	PRAL	fib	
TOTALS									

√	→	TO DO & TASK LIST

Hour	Schedule

Events of the day: ....

DATE .... weight ....

cups of fluid:

Food eaten	cal	fat	pro	pot	pho	sod	PRAL	fib	
TOTALS									

√	→	TO DO & TASK LIST

Hour	Schedule

Events of the day: ....

....

....

....

DATE .... weight ....

cups of fluid:

Food eaten	cal	fat	pro	pot	pho	sod	PRAL	fib	
TOTALS									

√	→	TO DO & TASK LIST

Hour	Schedule

Events of the day: ....

DATE .... weight ....

cups of fluid:

Food eaten	cal	fat	pro	pot	pho	sod	PRAL	fib	
TOTALS									

√	→	TO DO & TASK LIST

Hour	Schedule

Events of the day: ....

....

....

....

DATE .... weight ....

cups of fluid:

Food eaten	cal	fat	pro	pot	pho	sod	PRAL	fib	
TOTALS									

√	→	TO DO & TASK LIST

Hour	Schedule

Events of the day: ....

DATE .... weight ....

cups of fluid:

Food eaten	cal	fat	pro	pot	pho	sod	PRAL	fib	
TOTALS									

√	→	TO DO & TASK LIST

Hour	Schedule

Events of the day: ....

DATE .... weight ....

cups of fluid:

Food eaten	cal	fat	pro	pot	pho	sod	PRAL	fib	
TOTALS									

√	→	TO DO & TASK LIST

Hour	Schedule

Events of the day: ....

DATE ________________ weight ________

cups of fluid:

Food eaten	cal	fat	pro	pot	pho	sod	PRAL	fib	
TOTALS									

√	→	TO DO & TASK LIST

Hour	Schedule

Events of the day: ________________

DATE .... weight ....

cups of fluid:

Food eaten	cal	fat	pro	pot	pho	sod	PRAL	fib	
TOTALS									

√	→	TO DO & TASK LIST

Hour	Schedule

Events of the day: ....

DATE .... weight ....

cups of fluid:

Food eaten	cal	fat	pro	pot	pho	sod	PRAL	fib	
TOTALS									

√	→	TO DO & TASK LIST

Hour	Schedule

Events of the day: ....

....

....

....

DATE .... weight ....

cups of fluid:

Food eaten	cal	fat	pro	pot	pho	sod	PRAL	fib	
TOTALS									

√	→	TO DO & TASK LIST

Hour	Schedule

Events of the day: ....

DATE .... weight ....

cups of fluid:

Food eaten	cal	fat	pro	pot	pho	sod	PRAL	fib	
TOTALS									

√	→	TO DO & TASK LIST

Hour	Schedule

Events of the day: ....

DATE

weight

cups of fluid:

Food eaten	cal	fat	pro	pot	pho	sod	PRAL	fib	
TOTALS									

√	→	TO DO & TASK LIST

Hour	Schedule

Events of the day:

DATE .... weight ....

cups of fluid:

Food eaten	cal	fat	pro	pot	pho	sod	PRAL	fib	
TOTALS									

√	→	TO DO & TASK LIST

Hour	Schedule

Events of the day: ....

DATE ____________ weight ________

cups of fluid:

Food eaten	cal	fat	pro	pot	pho	sod	PRAL	fib	
TOTALS									

√	→	TO DO & TASK LIST

Hour	Schedule

Events of the day: ____________

DATE .... weight ....

cups of fluid:

Food eaten	cal	fat	pro	pot	pho	sod	PRAL	fib	
TOTALS									

√	→	TO DO & TASK LIST

Hour	Schedule

Events of the day: ....

DATE .... weight ....

cups of fluid:

Food eaten	cal	fat	pro	pot	pho	sod	PRAL	fib	
TOTALS									

√	→	TO DO & TASK LIST

Hour	Schedule

Events of the day: ....

DATE .... weight ....

cups of fluid:

Food eaten	cal	fat	pro	pot	pho	sod	PRAL	fib	
TOTALS									

√	→	TO DO & TASK LIST

Hour	Schedule

Events of the day: ....

DATE .... weight ....

cups of fluid:

Food eaten	cal	fat	pro	pot	pho	sod	PRAL	fib	
TOTALS									

√	→	TO DO & TASK LIST

Hour	Schedule

Events of the day: ....

DATE .... weight ....

cups of fluid:

Food eaten	cal	fat	pro	pot	pho	sod	PRAL	fib	
TOTALS									

√	→	TO DO & TASK LIST

Hour	Schedule

Events of the day: ....

DATE .... weight ....

cups of fluid:

Food eaten	cal	fat	pro	pot	pho	sod	PRAL	fib	
TOTALS									

√	→	TO DO & TASK LIST

Hour	Schedule

Events of the day: ....

DATE .... weight ....

cups of fluid:

Food eaten	cal	fat	pro	pot	pho	sod	PRAL	fib	
TOTALS									

√	→	TO DO & TASK LIST

Hour	Schedule

Events of the day: ....

DATE .... weight ....

cups of fluid:

Food eaten	cal	fat	pro	pot	pho	sod	PRAL	fib	
TOTALS									

√	→	TO DO & TASK LIST

Hour	Schedule

Events of the day: ....

DATE .... weight ....

cups of fluid:

Food eaten	cal	fat	pro	pot	pho	sod	PRAL	fib	
TOTALS									

√	→	TO DO & TASK LIST

Hour	Schedule

Events of the day: ....

....

....

....

DATE .... weight ....

cups of fluid:

Food eaten	cal	fat	pro	pot	pho	sod	PRAL	fib	
TOTALS									

√	→	TO DO & TASK LIST

Hour	Schedule

Events of the day: ....

DATE .... weight ....

cups of fluid:

Food eaten	cal	fat	pro	pot	pho	sod	PRAL	fib	
TOTALS									

√	→	TO DO & TASK LIST

Hour	Schedule

Events of the day: ....

DATE .... weight ....

cups of fluid:

Food eaten	cal	fat	pro	pot	pho	sod	PRAL	fib	
TOTALS									

√	→	TO DO & TASK LIST

Hour	Schedule

Events of the day: ....

....

....

....

DATE .... weight ....

cups of fluid:

Food eaten	cal	fat	pro	pot	pho	sod	PRAL	fib	
TOTALS									

√	→	TO DO & TASK LIST

Hour	Schedule

Events of the day: ....

....

....

....

DATE ....

weight ....

cups of fluid:

Food eaten	cal	fat	pro	pot	pho	sod	PRAL	fib	
TOTALS									

✓	→	TO DO & TASK LIST

Hour	Schedule

Events of the day: ....

DATE .... weight ....

cups of fluid:

Food eaten	cal	fat	pro	pot	pho	sod	PRAL	fib	
TOTALS									

√	→	TO DO & TASK LIST

Hour	Schedule

Events of the day: ....

DATE .... weight ....

cups of fluid:

Food eaten	cal	fat	pro	pot	pho	sod	PRAL	fib	
TOTALS									

√	→	TO DO & TASK LIST

Hour	Schedule

Events of the day: ....

DATE .... weight ....

cups of fluid:

Food eaten	cal	fat	pro	pot	pho	sod	PRAL	fib	
TOTALS									

√	→	TO DO & TASK LIST

Hour	Schedule

Events of the day: ....

DATE .... weight ....

cups of fluid:

Food eaten	cal	fat	pro	pot	pho	sod	PRAL	fib	
TOTALS									

√	→	TO DO & TASK LIST

Hour	Schedule

Events of the day: ....

DATE .... weight ....

cups of fluid:

Food eaten	cal	fat	pro	pot	pho	sod	PRAL	fib	
TOTALS									

√	→	TO DO & TASK LIST

Hour	Schedule

Events of the day: ....

DATE .... weight ....

cups of fluid:

Food eaten	cal	fat	pro	pot	pho	sod	PRAL	fib	
TOTALS									

√	→	TO DO & TASK LIST

Hour	Schedule

Events of the day: ....

DATE .... weight ....

cups of fluid:

Food eaten	cal	fat	pro	pot	pho	sod	PRAL	fib	
TOTALS									

√	→	TO DO & TASK LIST

Hour	Schedule

Events of the day: ....

DATE .... weight ....

cups of fluid:

Food eaten	cal	fat	pro	pot	pho	sod	PRAL	fib	
TOTALS									

√	→	TO DO & TASK LIST

Hour	Schedule

Events of the day: ....

....

....

....

DATE .... weight ....

cups of fluid:

Food eaten	cal	fat	pro	pot	pho	sod	PRAL	fib	
TOTALS									

√	→	TO DO & TASK LIST

Hour	Schedule

Events of the day: ....

....

....

....

DATE .... weight ....

cups of fluid:

Food eaten	cal	fat	pro	pot	pho	sod	PRAL	fib	
TOTALS									

√	→	TO DO & TASK LIST

Hour	Schedule

Events of the day: ....

DATE .... weight ....

cups of fluid:

Food eaten	cal	fat	pro	pot	pho	sod	PRAL	fib	
TOTALS									

√	→	TO DO & TASK LIST

Hour	Schedule

Events of the day: ....

DATE .... weight ....

cups of fluid:

Food eaten	cal	fat	pro	pot	pho	sod	PRAL	fib	
TOTALS									

√	→	TO DO & TASK LIST

Hour	Schedule

Events of the day: ....

DATE .... weight ....

cups of fluid:

Food eaten	cal	fat	pro	pot	pho	sod	PRAL	fib	
TOTALS									

√	→	TO DO & TASK LIST

Hour	Schedule

Events of the day: ....

DATE .... weight ....

cups of fluid:

Food eaten	cal	fat	pro	pot	pho	sod	PRAL	fib	
TOTALS									

√	→	TO DO & TASK LIST

Hour	Schedule

Events of the day: ....

....

....

....

DATE .... weight ....

cups of fluid:

Food eaten	cal	fat	pro	pot	pho	sod	PRAL	fib	
TOTALS									

√	→	TO DO & TASK LIST

Hour	Schedule

Events of the day: ....

....

....

....

DATE .... weight ....

cups of fluid:

Food eaten	cal	fat	pro	pot	pho	sod	PRAL	fib	
TOTALS									

√	→	TO DO & TASK LIST

Hour	Schedule

Events of the day: ....

DATE .... weight ....

cups of fluid:

Food eaten	cal	fat	pro	pot	pho	sod	PRAL	fib	
TOTALS									

√	→	TO DO & TASK LIST

Hour	Schedule

Events of the day: ....

DATE .... weight ....

cups of fluid:

Food eaten	cal	fat	pro	pot	pho	sod	PRAL	fib	
TOTALS									

√	→	TO DO & TASK LIST

Hour	Schedule

Events of the day: ....

....

....

....

DATE .... weight ....

cups of fluid:

Food eaten	cal	fat	pro	pot	pho	sod	PRAL	fib	
TOTALS									

√	→	TO DO & TASK LIST

Hour	Schedule

Events of the day: ....

....

....

....

DATE .... weight ....

cups of fluid:

Food eaten	cal	fat	pro	pot	pho	sod	PRAL	fib	
TOTALS									

√	→	TO DO & TASK LIST

Hour	Schedule

Events of the day: ....

....

....

....

DATE .... weight ....

cups of fluid:

Food eaten	cal	fat	pro	pot	pho	sod	PRAL	fib	
TOTALS									

√	→	TO DO & TASK LIST

Hour	Schedule

Events of the day: ....

DATE .... weight ....

cups of fluid:

Food eaten	cal	fat	pro	pot	pho	sod	PRAL	fib	
TOTALS									

√	→	TO DO & TASK LIST

Hour	Schedule

Events of the day: ....

DATE .... weight ....

cups of fluid:

Food eaten	cal	fat	pro	pot	pho	sod	PRAL	fib	
TOTALS									

√	→	TO DO & TASK LIST

Hour	Schedule

Events of the day: ....

DATE .... weight ....

cups of fluid:

Food eaten	cal	fat	pro	pot	pho	sod	PRAL	fib	
TOTALS									

√	→	TO DO & TASK LIST

Hour	Schedule

Events of the day: ....

....

....

....

DATE .... weight ....

cups of fluid:

Food eaten	cal	fat	pro	pot	pho	sod	PRAL	fib	
TOTALS									

√	→	TO DO & TASK LIST

Hour	Schedule

Events of the day: ....

DATE .... weight ....

cups of fluid:

Food eaten	cal	fat	pro	pot	pho	sod	PRAL	fib	
TOTALS									

√	→	TO DO & TASK LIST

Hour	Schedule

Events of the day: ....

DATE .... weight ....

cups of fluid:

Food eaten	cal	fat	pro	pot	pho	sod	PRAL	fib	
TOTALS									

√	→	TO DO & TASK LIST

Hour	Schedule

Events of the day: ....

DATE ________________ weight ________

cups of fluid:

Food eaten	cal	fat	pro	pot	pho	sod	PRAL	fib	
TOTALS									

√	→	TO DO & TASK LIST

Hour	Schedule

Events of the day: ________________

DATE .... weight ....

cups of fluid:

Food eaten	cal	fat	pro	pot	pho	sod	PRAL	fib	
TOTALS									

√	→	TO DO & TASK LIST

Hour	Schedule

Events of the day: ....

....

....

....

DATE .... weight ....

cups of fluid:

Food eaten	cal	fat	pro	pot	pho	sod	PRAL	fib	
TOTALS									

√	→	TO DO & TASK LIST

Hour	Schedule

Events of the day: ....

....

....

....

DATE .... weight ....

cups of fluid:

Food eaten	cal	fat	pro	pot	pho	sod	PRAL	fib	
TOTALS									

√	→	TO DO & TASK LIST

Hour	Schedule

Events of the day: ....

DATE .... weight ....

cups of fluid:

Food eaten	cal	fat	pro	pot	pho	sod	PRAL	fib	
TOTALS									

√	→	TO DO & TASK LIST

Hour	Schedule

Events of the day: ....

DATE .... weight ....

cups of fluid:

Food eaten	cal	fat	pro	pot	pho	sod	PRAL	fib	
TOTALS									

√	→	TO DO & TASK LIST

Hour	Schedule

Events of the day: ....

DATE .... weight ....

cups of fluid:

Food eaten	cal	fat	pro	pot	pho	sod	PRAL	fib	
TOTALS									

√	→	TO DO & TASK LIST

Hour	Schedule

Events of the day: ....

DATE .... weight ....

cups of fluid:

Food eaten	cal	fat	pro	pot	pho	sod	PRAL	fib	
TOTALS									

√	→	TO DO & TASK LIST

Hour	Schedule

Events of the day: ....

DATE .... weight ....

cups of fluid:

Food eaten	cal	fat	pro	pot	pho	sod	PRAL	fib	
TOTALS									

√	→	TO DO & TASK LIST

Hour	Schedule

Events of the day: ....

DATE .... weight ....

cups of fluid:

Food eaten	cal	fat	pro	pot	pho	sod	PRAL	fib	
TOTALS									

√	→	TO DO & TASK LIST

Hour	Schedule

Events of the day: ....

DATE .... weight ....

cups of fluid:

Food eaten	cal	fat	pro	pot	pho	sod	PRAL	fib	
TOTALS									

√	→	TO DO & TASK LIST

Hour	Schedule

Events of the day: ....

DATE .... weight ....

cups of fluid:

Food eaten	cal	fat	pro	pot	pho	sod	PRAL	fib	
TOTALS									

√	→	TO DO & TASK LIST

Hour	Schedule

Events of the day: ....

DATE .... weight ....

cups of fluid:

Food eaten	cal	fat	pro	pot	pho	sod	PRAL	fib	
TOTALS									

√	→	TO DO & TASK LIST

Hour	Schedule

Events of the day: ....

DATE .... weight ....

cups of fluid:

Food eaten	cal	fat	pro	pot	pho	sod	PRAL	fib	
TOTALS									

√	→	TO DO & TASK LIST

Hour	Schedule

Events of the day: ....

....

....

....

DATE .... weight ....

cups of fluid:

Food eaten	cal	fat	pro	pot	pho	sod	PRAL	fib	
TOTALS									

√	→	TO DO & TASK LIST

Hour	Schedule

Events of the day: ....

DATE .... weight ....

cups of fluid:

Food eaten	cal	fat	pro	pot	pho	sod	PRAL	fib	
TOTALS									

√	→	TO DO & TASK LIST

Hour	Schedule

Events of the day: ....

....

....

....

DATE .... weight ....

cups of fluid:

Food eaten	cal	fat	pro	pot	pho	sod	PRAL	fib	
TOTALS									

√	→	TO DO & TASK LIST

Hour	Schedule

Events of the day: ....

DATE .... weight ....

cups of fluid:

Food eaten	cal	fat	pro	pot	pho	sod	PRAL	fib	
TOTALS									

√	→	TO DO & TASK LIST

Hour	Schedule

Events of the day: ....

DATE .... weight ....

cups of fluid:

Food eaten	cal	fat	pro	pot	pho	sod	PRAL	fib	
TOTALS									

√	→	TO DO & TASK LIST

Hour	Schedule

Events of the day: ....

DATE .... weight ....

cups of fluid:

Food eaten	cal	fat	pro	pot	pho	sod	PRAL	fib	
TOTALS									

√	→	TO DO & TASK LIST

Hour	Schedule

Events of the day: ....

DATE .... weight ....

cups of fluid:

Food eaten	cal	fat	pro	pot	pho	sod	PRAL	fib	
TOTALS									

√	→	TO DO & TASK LIST

Hour	Schedule

Events of the day: ....

DATE ______________________ weight ____________

cups of fluid:

Food eaten	cal	fat	pro	pot	pho	sod	PRAL	fib	
TOTALS									

√	→	TO DO & TASK LIST

Hour	Schedule

Events of the day: ____

____

____

____

DATE .... weight ....

cups of fluid:

Food eaten	cal	fat	pro	pot	pho	sod	PRAL	fib	
TOTALS									

√	→	TO DO & TASK LIST

Hour	Schedule

Events of the day: ....

DATE

weight

cups of fluid:

Food eaten	cal	fat	pro	pot	pho	sod	PRAL	fib	
TOTALS									

√	→	TO DO & TASK LIST

Hour	Schedule

Events of the day:

DATE .... weight ....

cups of fluid:

Food eaten	cal	fat	pro	pot	pho	sod	PRAL	fib	
TOTALS									

√	→	TO DO & TASK LIST

Hour	Schedule

Events of the day: ....

....

....

....

DATE .... weight ....

cups of fluid:

Food eaten	cal	fat	pro	pot	pho	sod	PRAL	fib	
TOTALS									

√	→	TO DO & TASK LIST

Hour	Schedule

Events of the day: ....

DATE .... weight ....

cups of fluid:

Food eaten	cal	fat	pro	pot	pho	sod	PRAL	fib	
TOTALS									

√	→	TO DO & TASK LIST

Hour	Schedule

Events of the day: ....

DATE .... weight ....

cups of fluid:

Food eaten	cal	fat	pro	pot	pho	sod	PRAL	fib	
TOTALS									

√	→	TO DO & TASK LIST

Hour	Schedule

Events of the day: ....

DATE .... weight ....

cups of fluid:

Food eaten	cal	fat	pro	pot	pho	sod	PRAL	fib	
TOTALS									

√	→	TO DO & TASK LIST

Hour	Schedule

Events of the day: ....

DATE .... weight ....

cups of fluid:

Food eaten	cal	fat	pro	pot	pho	sod	PRAL	fib	
TOTALS									

√	→	TO DO & TASK LIST

Hour	Schedule

Events of the day: ....

....

....

....

DATE .... weight ....

cups of fluid:

Food eaten	cal	fat	pro	pot	pho	sod	PRAL	fib	
TOTALS									

√	→	TO DO & TASK LIST

Hour	Schedule

Events of the day: ....

DATE ____________ weight ________

cups of fluid:

Food eaten	cal	fat	pro	pot	pho	sod	PRAL	fib	
TOTALS									

√	→	TO DO & TASK LIST

Hour	Schedule

Events of the day: ____________

DATE .... weight ....

cups of fluid:

Food eaten	cal	fat	pro	pot	pho	sod	PRAL	fib	
TOTALS									

√	→	TO DO & TASK LIST

Hour	Schedule

Events of the day: ....

....

....

....

DATE .... weight ....

cups of fluid:

Food eaten	cal	fat	pro	pot	pho	sod	PRAL	fib	
TOTALS									

√	→	TO DO & TASK LIST

Hour	Schedule

Events of the day: ....

DATE .... weight ....

cups of fluid:

Food eaten	cal	fat	pro	pot	pho	sod	PRAL	fib	
TOTALS									

√	→	TO DO & TASK LIST

Hour	Schedule

Events of the day: ....

DATE .... weight ....

cups of fluid:

Food eaten	cal	fat	pro	pot	pho	sod	PRAL	fib	
TOTALS									

√	→	TO DO & TASK LIST

Hour	Schedule

Events of the day: ....

....

....

....

DATE .... weight ....

cups of fluid:

Food eaten	cal	fat	pro	pot	pho	sod	PRAL	fib	
TOTALS									

√	→	TO DO & TASK LIST

Hour	Schedule

Events of the day: ....

DATE .... weight ....

cups of fluid:

Food eaten	cal	fat	pro	pot	pho	sod	PRAL	fib	
TOTALS									

√	→	TO DO & TASK LIST

Hour	Schedule

Events of the day: ....

DATE .... weight ....

cups of fluid:

Food eaten	cal	fat	pro	pot	pho	sod	PRAL	fib	
TOTALS									

√	→	TO DO & TASK LIST

Hour	Schedule

Events of the day: ....

DATE ______________________ weight ______________

cups of fluid:

Food eaten	cal	fat	pro	pot	pho	sod	PRAL	fib	
TOTALS									

√	→	TO DO & TASK LIST

Hour	Schedule

Events of the day: ____

DATE .... weight ....

cups of fluid:

Food eaten	cal	fat	pro	pot	pho	sod	PRAL	fib	
TOTALS									

√	→	TO DO & TASK LIST

Hour	Schedule

Events of the day: ....

DATE .... weight ....

cups of fluid:

Food eaten	cal	fat	pro	pot	pho	sod	PRAL	fib	
TOTALS									

√	→	TO DO & TASK LIST

Hour	Schedule

Events of the day: ....

....

....

....

DATE .... weight ....

cups of fluid:

Food eaten	cal	fat	pro	pot	pho	sod	PRAL	fib	
TOTALS									

√	→	TO DO & TASK LIST

Hour	Schedule

Events of the day: ....

DATE .... weight ....

cups of fluid:

Food eaten	cal	fat	pro	pot	pho	sod	PRAL	fib	
TOTALS									

√	→	TO DO & TASK LIST

Hour	Schedule

Events of the day: ....

DATE .... weight ....

cups of fluid:

Food eaten	cal	fat	pro	pot	pho	sod	PRAL	fib	
TOTALS									

√	→	TO DO & TASK LIST

Hour	Schedule

Events of the day: ....

DATE .... weight ....

cups of fluid:

Food eaten	cal	fat	pro	pot	pho	sod	PRAL	fib	
TOTALS									

√	→	TO DO & TASK LIST

Hour	Schedule

Events of the day: ....

DATE .... weight ....

cups of fluid:

Food eaten	cal	fat	pro	pot	pho	sod	PRAL	fib	
TOTALS									

√	→	TO DO & TASK LIST

Hour	Schedule

Events of the day: ....

FOOD VALUE LIST, LABS, NOTES

FOOD VALUE LIST, LABS, NOTES

FOOD VALUE LIST, LABS, NOTES

FOOD VALUE LIST, LABS, NOTES

FOOD VALUE LIST, LABS, NOTES

FOOD VALUE LIST, LABS, NOTES

FOOD VALUE LIST, LABS, NOTES

FOOD VALUE LIST, LABS, NOTES

FOOD VALUE LIST, LABS, NOTES

FOOD VALUE LIST, LABS, NOTES

Made in the USA
Monee, IL
20 April 2026

48663217R00118